HERBAL REMEDIES FOR BLOOD DETOXIFICATION

Harnessing The Power Of Herbs For Natural Body Nourishment, Cleansing, Rejuvenating, And Lifestyle Changes For Optimal Well-Being

DR. CARDEN KYRIE

DISCLAIMER

The only goal of this book is informational. Every effort has been taken by the author and publisher to ensure that the information provided is accurate. But the material in this book is given "as is," without any express or implied representation, warranty, or condition as to its accuracy, completeness, or suitability for any particular purpose.

Any loss, damage, or injury resulting from using the information in this book, or from any action or decision made as a result of such use, will not be covered by the author's or publisher's liability. It is recommended that readers seek the assistance of a certified specialist for guidance specific to their situation.

The opinions and viewpoints conveyed in this book belong to the author and may not necessarily represent the official stance or policies of any specified organizations or people. Any likeness to real-life occurrences, places, or people—living or deceased—is wholly coincidental.

No specific product, service, or therapy discussed in this book is endorsed by the author or publisher. Any reference to goods or services is made only for informative reasons and is not intended as a recommendation or endorsement.

Before making any judgments or acting on any information, readers are urged to independently confirm it all. Any unfavorable effects or repercussions arising from the usage of the material included in this book are disclaimed by the author and publisher.

By using this book, you consent to absolving the publisher and author of any and all claims, obligations, or losses resulting from your use of the material in it.

I appreciate your cooperation and understanding.

TABLE OF CONTENTS

INTRODUCTION TO BLOOD DETOXIFICATION

THE SIGNIFICANCE OF DETOXIFYING BLOOD

An essential function of the human body that is critical to preserving general health and well-being is blood cleansing. The process's importance arises from its capacity to remove waste materials, toxic compounds, and poisons from the bloodstream, hence guaranteeing the appropriate operation of essential organs and systems. Because the bloodstream is the body's lifeline, carrying hormones, nutrition, and oxygen to all areas of the body, it must be kept free of harmful substances that could impair its effectiveness. Blood detoxification is crucial for more reasons than just clearing the circulatory system; it also affects the body's metabolism, immune system, and general ability to fend off illness.

Herbal therapies are one way to effectively achieve blood detoxification, which is different from traditional pharmacological interventions. The rich history of natural medicine is the foundation of herbal approaches to blood detoxification, which rely on the medicinal qualities of many different plants to enhance the body's natural detoxification processes. By treating the underlying causes of toxicity and reducing the possibility of harmful side effects that are frequently connected with synthetic medications, these herbal remedies provide a gentle and comprehensive approach to blood purification. To fully appreciate the all-encompassing character of herbal treatments in promoting blood health, one must have a thorough understanding of the wide variety of herbs and their unique detoxifying abilities.

AN OVERVIEW OF HERBAL REMEDIES

Herbal methods of blood detoxification include a broad spectrum of plant-based treatments that have been used for ages in many traditional medical systems around the world. These particular biochemical characteristics of these herbs boost liver function, improve renal filtration, and facilitate waste product removal, which is why they were selected. In particular, the liver is crucial to blood detoxification because it processes and neutralizes toxins. Many herbs include hepatoprotective properties that support the liver's vital roles. Herbs with diuretic qualities can also increase kidney function, encouraging waste to be excreted through urine and aiding in the bloodstream's general cleaning.

Knowing the significance of blood detoxification sheds light on the vital function it plays in preserving optimum health. Herbal remedies recognize the interdependence of many body systems and provide a natural, comprehensive way to assist the body's natural detoxification processes. When we examine the overview of herbal treatments, we find that they offer a complex and multidimensional approach to supporting blood health, which is a reflection of the knowledge gathered over centuries of traditional medical practices.

CHAPTER ONE

COMPREHENDING BLOOD DETOXIFICATION

BLOOD'S FUNCTION IN THE BODY

The blood is an essential connective tissue that carries waste products, nutrition, hormones, and oxygen to and from different cells and organs in the human body. Blood is made up of platelets, plasma, and red and white blood cells, and flows via an intricate system of vessels to support the body's functions. It functions as a dynamic medium that makes it easier for various bodily parts to communicate with one another, promoting general health and balance.

THE VALUE OF BLOOD DETOXIFICATION

The significance of blood detoxification cannot be emphasized, given the vital function blood plays in maintaining life. To ensure that the bloodstream is operating at its best, detoxification is a necessary and natural process that helps remove dangerous toxins from the bloodstream. Toxin buildup in the blood can result in several health problems, such as weakened immune systems, inflammation, and abnormalities in metabolic functions. The body can better fend against illnesses, keep hormone levels in check, and promote the smooth operation of vital organs like the liver and kidneys by cleansing the blood.

TYPICAL TOXINS THAT IMPACT BLOOD HEALTH

Numerous everyday pollutants have the potential to negatively impact blood health, making cleansing necessary. Air, water, and food sources can all introduce environmental contaminants into the bloodstream, including heavy metals, pesticides, and industrial chemicals. Toxins in the blood can also be caused by lifestyle factors such as smoking, excessive alcohol intake, and bad food choices. The natural detoxification processes of the body, which are mostly handled by the liver, are designed to counteract and get rid of these dangerous toxins. But if the body can't eliminate all the toxins, it can accumulate these chemicals in the blood, which can be dangerous for general health.

Furthermore, waste chemicals and metabolic wastes produced by the body can potentially cause blood poisoning. Ineffective removal of metabolic waste can lead to the build-up of compounds such as creatinine and urea, which can be harmful to blood health if left unchecked. Physical and mental stress can increase the level of toxins in the blood by releasing stress hormones and impairing the body's capacity to properly detoxify.

Sustaining general health requires an awareness of the pollutants that commonly impair blood health, the function of blood in the body, and the significance of detoxification. A balanced diet, frequent exercise, and enough hydration are examples of healthy lifestyle choices that can assist the body's natural detoxification processes and advance ideal blood health.

CHAPTER TWO

FUNDAMENTALS OF COMPLEMENTARY MEDICINE

OVERVIEW OF HERBAL MEDICINE

Herbalism is a conventional medical practice that uses the therapeutic qualities of plants to enhance health and well-being. It is sometimes referred to as phytotherapy or botanical medicine. Herbalism has its roots in many ancient cultures and has developed over centuries, absorbing knowledge that has been passed down through the generations. Herbal medicine is based on the core idea that plants have medicinal properties that have beneficial effects on human health. Herbalism emphasizes the holistic synergy of the entire plant, in contrast to traditional medicine, which frequently isolates particular active compounds.

Since the beginning of time, people have utilized herbs as medicine, with many different civilizations depending on the natural world's knowledge to treat a range of health issues. Using this collection of knowledge, herbalists—those who practice herbal medicine—create treatments that aid in the body's innate healing abilities. Herbal medicine is more than just treating symptoms; it's about realizing how intertwined mental, emotional, and spiritual health are. Given that every person reacts differently to plant-based therapies, herbalism promotes a customized strategy.

THE EFFECTS OF HERBS ON THE BODY

Investigating the intricate relationships that exist between plant chemicals and human physiology is necessary to comprehend how herbs function in the body. Numerous bioactive substances found in herbs, such as polyphenols, alkaloids, flavonoids, and essential oils, contribute to their therapeutic qualities. These substances interact with the body's systems, affecting metabolic reactions and encouraging equilibrium.

The idea of adaptogens herbs that assist the body in adjusting to stress and preserving homeostasis is a fundamental component of herbal medicine. Herbs known to be adaptogenic, such as ashwagandha and ginseng, influence how the body reacts to stimuli and promote resilience in general. Furthermore, depending on their components, herbs may have antibacterial, anti-inflammatory, or antioxidant properties. Herbalism's holistic approach recognizes that the human body is a dynamic, linked system and that there are many different ways in which herbs interact with it.

Herbs can influence several body systems, such as the immunological, circulatory, and neurological systems. Herbs that are known to relax the nervous system, such as valerian and chamomile, can help reduce tension and anxiety. Herbs that promote circulation and control blood pressure, like garlic and hawthorn, may help with heart health. Herbal therapy acknowledges that by carefully selecting herbs, the body's natural capacity for self-healing can be strengthened and encouraged.

SELECTING THE OPTIMAL HERBS FOR PURIFICATION

The goal of detoxification is to improve the body's inherent detoxification processes and remove toxins from the body. In herbal treatment, knowing the unique requirements of the patient as well as the organs or systems being detoxified is crucial to choosing the appropriate herbs. Herbs can aid in detoxification in several ways, such as by promoting kidney and liver function and stimulating the lymphatic system.

One well-known plant that helps with liver function and cleansing is milk thistle. It includes silymarin, an antioxidant-rich substance that may shield liver cells from harm and facilitate the removal of pollutants. Another herb with diuretic qualities is dandelion root, which enhances kidney function and encourages waste materials to be eliminated by urine.

Combinations of plants having diuretic, laxative, and cholagogue (increasing bile flow) qualities are frequently found in herbal mixes intended for detoxification. This synergistic method guarantees a gentle and balanced detoxification process while aiding in the removal of pollutants from the body. Herbs that are frequently used for detoxification include cleavers, burdock root, and nettle, which are thought to help the lymphatic system.

The foundational ideas of herbal therapy contain a comprehensive comprehension of the interrelationship between plants and the human anatomy. Herbalism acknowledges the complex ways in which plants affect physiological processes to support health and well-being by interacting with the body's systems. In terms of detoxification, the thoughtful selection of herbs based on a person's specific requirements can support the body's inherent capacity to get rid of toxins, promoting a harmonious and balanced state of being.

CHAPTER THREE

HERBS FOR BLOOD CLEANSING

DANDELION ROOT

Because of its potential to assist blood detoxification, dandelion root, scientifically known as Taraxacum officinale, has long been employed in herbal therapy. Dandelion root, which is high in antioxidants, is thought to aid the liver in removing toxins from the blood. Its anti-inflammatory qualities are attributed to the presence of substances like flavonoids and polyphenols, which support general detoxifying procedures.

BURDOCK ROOT

The Arctium lappa plant yields burdock root, which is prized for its blood-purifying qualities. It has active ingredients such as polyacetylenes, flavonoids, and inulin that are believed to enhance liver function and encourage the removal of toxins from the bloodstream.

Burdock root's diuretic properties may also aid in the elimination of waste by promoting the production of more urine.

TURMERIC

The spice with a golden tint that comes from the Curcuma longa plant has a strong anti-inflammatory and antioxidant ingredient called curcumin. Turmeric is widely known for its anti-inflammatory properties, but it's also thought to benefit liver function. Turmeric aids in the creation of enzymes that actively take part in detoxifying, which helps with the blood's general cleansing.

RED CLOVER

Known for its estrogen-like properties, Red Clover (Trifolium pratense) is a flowering plant that is high in isoflavones. This plant is said to help the lymphatic system, which improves the blood's ability to eliminate waste and pollutants. Red clover's ability to aid in blood cleansing may also be influenced by its possible diuretic properties.

MILK THISTLE

The active ingredient silymarin is mostly responsible for the hepatoprotective qualities of milk thistle (Silybum marianum). This herb is believed to help the liver by encouraging the regeneration of liver cells and improving the liver's capacity for detoxification. In cleansing regimens, milk thistle is frequently utilized as a supporting plant.

ECHINACEA

Echinacea, which comes from the Echinacea purpurea plant, is frequently linked to the maintenance of the immune system. But its ability to promote the development of white blood cells which are essential for eliminating toxins and infections from the bloodstream underpins its possible involvement in blood detoxification. The immune-stimulating properties of echinacea may indirectly aid in general detoxification.

ALLIUM SATIVUM

Allium sativum, or garlic, has been used for a very long time for a variety of health advantages, including the possibility that it could improve cardiovascular health. Garlic has a sulfur-containing chemical called allicin, which may have detoxifying effects. Garlic may enhance the liver's detoxification activities and help remove heavy metals from the blood.

GINGER

Zingiber officinale, or ginger, is highly valued for its antioxidant and anti-inflammatory qualities. Ginger has long been associated with digestive health advantages, but it may also aid in blood detoxification. Some of its key ingredients, like gingerol, have been researched for their ability to improve the body's natural detoxification processes and promote liver function.

CHAPTER FOUR

HERBAL TEA INFUSIONS FOR PURIFYING THE BLOOD

HERBAL TEA RECIPES FOR DETOXIFICATION

Carefully choosing plants with detoxifying qualities is necessary when blending herbal teas for blood purification. Dandelion root is a common option since it is thought to support the removal of toxins from the bloodstream and stimulate liver function. When combined with burdock root, which is well known for its blood-purifying properties, it can help accelerate the process of detoxification. Nettle leaf is an additional beneficial supplement since it helps the kidneys and aids in the body's elimination of waste and pollutants.

It can be calming to the taste and helpful for digestion to give a hint of calming flavor to the mixture by adding chamomile or mint leaves. These herbs not only improve the flavor but also offer extra health advantages, which add to the enjoyment of the cleansing process. It's crucial to test out various ratios to identify the ideal combination that maximizes each herb's health advantages while accommodating personal tastes.

DIRECTIONS FOR BREWING AND CONSUMPTION

The right methods for preparing and drinking herbal tea blends are essential to their efficacy in purifying the blood. It is best to use hot water that is just below boiling to extract the maximum amount of medicinal components from the plants. After allowing the water to absorb the active ingredients, steeping the herbs for five to ten minutes results in a strong and tasty brew.

To have a smoother texture and a more pleasurable drinking experience, straining the tea after steeping is essential for removing any herbal particles. A spoonful of honey or a splash of lemon can improve the flavor and offer extra cleansing advantages for individuals who like a little sweetness. When the herbal tea is had early in the morning or right before bed, the body is better able to absorb the nutrients and initiate the detoxification process.

INCLUDING HERBAL TEAS IN EVERYDAY ACTIVITIES

Herbal teas should be included in a regular blood cleansing regimen with consistency and attentiveness. Start by switching to a cup of the detoxifying herbal blend for one of the normal teas or coffees. By introducing the new regimen gradually, the body can get used to it without being overtaxed.

Think about introducing herbal teas into particular times of the day, like an afternoon or mid-morning ritual, to establish a deliberate break in the regular schedule. This promotes calmness and guarantees that the herbal blend's cleansing properties are routinely incorporated into the daily routine. Carrying a thermos of herbal tea with you all day promotes staying hydrated and gives you an easy way to routinely drink the cleansing infusion.

The process of creating herbal tea blends for blood cleaning necessitates a careful selection of detoxifying herbs, and the methods for brewing and consuming them are critical to optimizing their medicinal properties. Consistency and attention are necessary when incorporating these teas into daily life to facilitate a smooth transition to a healthy way of living.

CHAPTER FIVE

METHODS OF LIVING FOR BLOOD DETOXIFICATION

A BALANCED DIET FOR PURIFYING THE BLOOD

A balanced diet is fundamental to general health and plays a major role in blood purification. Nutrient-dense foods can help the body's natural detoxification processes; just include them in your daily meals. Fresh produce aids in the removal of toxins from the circulation, especially antioxidant-rich foods like kale, spinach, and berries. Furthermore, adding ginger, garlic, and turmeric to the diet helps improve liver function a crucial organ in the detoxification of the blood.

THE EFFECTS OF EXERCISE ON BLOOD HEALTH

Exercise regularly is essential for preserving ideal blood health. Exercise increases circulation, which facilitates the body's effective delivery of nutrients and oxygen.

Cardiovascular workouts, including running, cycling, or brisk walking, enhance blood flow and stimulate the heart, which helps the body eliminate waste. In addition to improving general fitness, strength training activities help the body maintain a healthy weight and control blood sugar levels, two processes that are directly related to blood detoxification.

TECHNIQUES FOR REDUCING STRESS

Techniques for reducing stress are essential for assisting with blood cleansing. Persistent stress can impair the body's capacity to expel toxins, which can result in a buildup of dangerous compounds in the blood. Deep breathing techniques, yoga, and mindfulness meditation have all been demonstrated to lower stress and increase relaxation. People who are good at managing stress have a favorable impact on their hormonal balance, which in turn helps the body's natural detoxifying processes.

HYDRATION AND DETOXIFICATION OF THE BLOOD

One essential component of blood detoxification is hydration. Water is essential for the body's detoxification processes, which include perspiration and urine. Maintaining proper hydration is essential for the kidneys, which are in charge of filtering and eliminating waste. Drinking herbal teas, infusing water, and eating foods high in water content, such as cucumbers and watermelon, can also help the body stay hydrated overall and aid in the detoxification process.

Reducing alcohol and sugary drink use is also crucial since these substances can put stress on the liver and make it more difficult for it to properly cleanse the blood.

A lifestyle centered around a diet high in nutrients, consistent exercise, managing stress, and maintaining adequate hydration may greatly aid in the process of blood detoxification.

Together, these techniques assist the body's natural detoxification processes, enhancing general health and vigor. Through the integration of these routines into their daily lives, people may cultivate a comprehensive perspective on blood health and augment their general welfare.

CHAPTER SIX

PROGRAMS FOR DETOXIFICATION AND CLEANSES

SYNOPSIS OF DETOX INITIATIVES

Programs and cleanses for detoxification have grown in popularity as more individuals look for solutions to improve their health and well-being. The main goals of these regimens are usually to detoxify the body, improve general health, and give the system a new lease of life. Although the idea of detoxification has been present for millennia in many traditional and cultural traditions, contemporary detox regimens sometimes include particular treatments, dietary modifications, and lifestyle alterations.

FORMULATING A CUSTOMIZED DETOX PROGRAM

Developing an individualized detox strategy is essential to maximizing the efficacy of these programs. When it comes to detoxification, there is no one-size-fits-all solution because there are several variables to consider, including age, health, and specific health objectives. A customized strategy takes into account each person's physiology, food choices, and way of life, customizing the detox regimen to suit their requirements. The length of the detox, the kinds of meals consumed, and the addition of extra activities like exercise or meditation are all crucial components in designing a plan that supports a person's objectives and general well-being.

WARNINGS AND THINGS TO THINK ABOUT

People should take a few safety measures and factors into account before starting a detox program. Before beginning any detox program, it is imperative to speak with a healthcare provider, particularly for people who are on medication or have pre-existing medical issues. Detox programs, which include abrupt and significant changes, can have various impacts on different people. Seeking expert advice can help ensure that the procedure is safe and appropriate for a person's particular health situation.

People should also be cautious about excessive or unduly restricted detox treatments that offer instant results. Quick weight reduction or extreme detoxification procedures might result in dietary shortages and other unfavorable health effects. In general, a steady and balanced approach is more maintainable and less likely to result in negative reactions. Keeping yourself well hydrated is also crucial during a detox since more fluids aid in the body's natural removal processes.

People should also be aware of any possible detox symptoms. Some people may have symptoms including headaches, exhaustion, or changes in bowel patterns while the body gets rid of pollutants. It's important to listen to your body and modify the detox plan as necessary, even though these symptoms are usually transient and an indication that your body is changing.

A healthcare provider should be consulted if symptoms become severe or persistent.

When used thoughtfully and with customized planning, detoxification regimens and cleanses may be effective instruments for enhancing general health and well-being. A safe and successful detoxification process requires knowing the unique nature of detox, speaking with medical specialists, and being aware of potential safety measures.

CHAPTER SEVEN

SAFETY AND PRECAUTIONS
RECOGNIZING POSSIBLE DANGERS

A complete awareness of potential hazards is essential to safety and safeguards in any undertaking linked to health. Before starting a detoxification journey, people should be informed about the possible drawbacks and difficulties that might occur. The body may react differently to different detoxification techniques, causing anything from little pain to more severe symptoms. People need to educate themselves on the particular detox process they are doing, taking into account things like how long it will take, how intense it will be, and how it can affect their general health.

Moreover, it is critical to acknowledge individual differences in detoxification response. For some people, a procedure that seems doable could provide difficulties. Pre-existing medical disorders, medicines, and general lifestyle choices can all have a big impact on how the body responds to the detoxification process. This emphasizes how crucial it is to use customized detoxification strategies and have a thorough awareness of one's unique health profile.

CONSULTATION WITH MEDICAL SPECIALISTS

Maintaining open lines of contact with medical specialists while pursuing a detoxification plan is an essential preventive step. Before beginning any detox program, people should speak with licensed healthcare providers, such as doctors or registered dietitians, who may offer individualized advice based on the patient's medical history, present circumstances, and desired outcomes.

Healthcare practitioners can customize advice to meet the specific needs of each patient and provide insightful information about the possible hazards connected with a certain detox procedure. They can also offer advice on the length and level of rigor of detox programs, making sure that they complement the person's general state of health. Throughout the detoxification process, this cooperative approach reduces possible health hazards and creates a foundation for wise decision-making.

KEEPING AN EYE ON AND MODIFYING DETOXIFICATION PLANS

Because the human body is dynamic, detoxification regimens must be constantly monitored and adjusted as needed. Vigilant introspection and frequent follow-ups with medical experts are crucial elements of a secure detoxification process. Keeping a tight eye on the body's reactions to the detoxification process includes monitoring any changes in mood, energy levels, digestion, or other physiological indicators.

Based on these findings and any advice given by medical specialists, modifications to detoxification programs could be necessary. Being adaptable is essential since people's reactions to detoxification techniques might change over time. Modifying the detox plan under the supervision of a healthcare provider can help prevent future health concerns and guarantee a more individualized and effective response in the event of bad reactions or unforeseen issues.

A safety-conscious approach to detoxification must include a thorough awareness of potential hazards, collaboration with medical specialists, and continual monitoring with the flexibility to modify detoxification strategies. People may approach detoxification with more confidence and reduce any potential health risks by emphasizing educated decision-making and customized treatment.

CHAPTER EIGHT

INCLUDING HERBAL DETOXIFICATION IN EVERYDAY ACTIVITIES

LONG-TERM BLOOD HEALTH STRATEGIES

Maintaining long-term blood health is an all-encompassing activity that requires a mix of dietary habits, cleansing routines, and lifestyle decisions. Keeping a nutritious, well-balanced diet that supports the body's natural detoxifying processes is a key component of sustaining blood health. Eating meals high in cruciferous vegetables, berries, and leafy greens can help remove toxins from the bloodstream by supplying vital vitamins and antioxidants.

Long-term blood health is greatly supported by adequate hydration. Getting enough water in your diet aids in toxin removal and enhances blood circulation. Herbal drinks with extra detoxifying properties, like dandelion or burdock root tea, can help with hydration even more. Maintaining enough hydration is essential to the body's natural detoxification processes.

A further essential component of long-term blood health is regular physical exercise. Improved blood circulation from exercise helps the body carry nutrients and oxygen more effectively throughout. Exercise-induced sweating aids in the skin's ability to remove toxins. Regularly participating in physical activities like yoga, running, or brisk walking improves the circulatory system's general health in addition to cardiovascular health.

Proper stress management is essential for maintaining long-term blood health. Prolonged stress can raise cortisol levels, which can damage the cardiovascular system and cause inflammation. Long-term support for good blood health may be obtained by integrating stress-reduction methods like deep breathing exercises, mindfulness, or meditation into everyday living. These practices can assist in maintaining a harmonic balance inside the body.

SUSTAINING A LIFESTYLE DETOX

A detoxified lifestyle is more than just quick cleanses; it's about making deliberate decisions every day. The emphasis on whole, nutrient-dense meals that assist the body's detoxifying processes is fundamental to this way of living. A diet high in antioxidants, fiber, and vital nutrients supplies the building blocks needed for the effective elimination of toxins from the blood.

In addition to nutritional concerns, reducing exposure to environmental pollutants is vital for keeping a detoxified lifestyle. This includes reducing the consumption of processed foods, limiting exposure to household chemicals, and choosing organic products whenever possible. Mindful consumption extends to personal care products, with a preference for natural and chemical-free options that support skin health and reduce the body's overall toxic burden.

Regular incorporation of herbal detoxifiers into daily routines further enhances the detoxification process.

Herbs such as milk thistle, turmeric, and cilantro have been traditionally recognized for their liver-supporting properties, assisting the body in breaking down and eliminating toxins. Integrating these herbs into meals, teas, or supplements can provide ongoing support for the body's natural detox mechanisms.

Creating a sleep routine that prioritizes adequate and quality sleep is a fundamental aspect of maintaining a detoxified lifestyle. During sleep, the body undergoes essential repair and regeneration processes, including the elimination of toxins from the brain and other tissues. Establishing consistent sleep patterns supports overall well-being and ensures that the body can effectively carry out its detoxification functions.

ADAPTING DETOX PRACTICES AS NEEDED

Flexibility in detox practices is essential, as individual needs and circumstances may change over time. Adapting detox practices involves staying attuned to the body's signals and adjusting routines accordingly. Periodic reassessment of dietary choices, stress management techniques, and herbal supplements allows for a personalized approach to detoxification.

Seasonal detox rituals can provide a structured framework for adapting detox practices throughout the year. Aligning dietary choices with seasonal, locally available produce and incorporating specific herbs that align with seasonal needs can optimize the body's ability to adapt to environmental changes. This approach acknowledges the dynamic nature of detoxification and emphasizes the importance of adjusting practices based on external and internal factors.

Listening to the body's responses to different detox strategies is paramount. While some individuals may benefit from more intensive detox protocols, others may find that gentler, ongoing practices better suit their needs. Paying attention to energy levels, digestive function, and overall well-being allows for a nuanced and responsive approach to adapting detox practices as needed.

Incorporating regular health check-ups and consultations with healthcare professionals is a crucial aspect of adapting detox practices. Professional guidance can help individuals tailor their detoxification strategies based on specific health conditions, ensuring a safe and effective approach. Collaboration with healthcare providers fosters a comprehensive understanding of individual health needs and promotes a proactive and informed stance toward adapting detox practices over time.